The Rockwool Foundation Research Unit

Children's health-related life-styles:
How parental child care affects them

Jens Bonke and Jane Greve

University Press of Southern Denmark
Odense 2013

**Children's health-related life-styles:
How parental child care affects them**

Discussion Paper

Published by:
© The Rockwool Foundation Research Unit and
University Press of Southern Denmark

Address:
The Rockwool Foundation Research Unit
Sølvgade 10
DK-1307 Copenhagen K

ISBN 978-87-90199-75-3
Print: Narayana Press

Price: 60.00 DKK, including 25% VAT

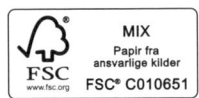

Contents

Abstract	5
1. Introduction	6
2. Data	8
3. The empirical strategy	11
4. Results	13
4.1 Parental working time and child care time	13
4.2 Parental working time and children's activities	14
4.3 Parental child care time and children's activities	16
4.4 Parental activities and child activities	17
5. Conclusions	20
References	22
Appendix	25

Children's health-related life-styles:
How parental child care affects them

Jens Bonke and Jane Greve

Abstract

This paper examines parental influence on school children's everyday activities that are related to a healthy or an unhealthy lifestyle. Using the Danish Time-Use and Consumption Survey (DTUC) from 2008/09 with information on fathers', mothers' and children's time use, we found no evidence of a relationship between parental working hours and children's time allocations, while a one-hour increase in parental child care reduces the time children spent on TV/computer games by 12 to 19 minutes. We also found a relationship between parents' and their children's time use, as the amounts of time the two generations spent on exercise were positively correlated, which indicates that parental time use on some healthy activities affects children's lifestyle behavior more than parental child care.

Keywords
Children's time use, children's lifestyles, parental working hours.

JEL Classification
I12, J22, D13

1. Introduction

Numerous studies have linked changes in eating habits and changes in time spent on physical activity and television viewing to the increasing prevalence of childhood obesity that almost all Western countries have experienced in the last 20-30 years (Ebbelin et al. 2002). Moreover, physical inactivity induces several negative effects on the cardiovascular system, skeletal muscle, bones and metabolism in adulthood (e.g. Kiens et al. 2007). A recent study (Bonke & Greve 2010) shows that 19-24% of Danish children aged 7 to 17 were overweight in 2010. The weight gains and current increases in obesity levels in both Denmark and most other Western countries have been shown to result from only a slight shift towards a positive energy balance, i.e. more energy in than energy out. Thus, most weight gains could be prevented with small behavioral changes, such as increased physical activity, small decreases in dietary fat or sugar intake and smaller portion sizes (Cutler et al. 2003, Lean et al. 2006).

In the framework of a simple economic model obesity is considered a function of an individual's energy balance, defined as caloric intake minus energy expenditure, over a number of time periods, and individual specific variables measuring, e.g. age, gender, ethnicity and genetic predisposition for obesity (Chou et al. 2002). When extending this economic framework to children, one must take into account that children are to some extent limited in their choices by their parents' choices and limitations.[1] In the child health production function the main input is parents' time with their children. Assuming that parents are those who are best at taking care of their children, the benefits of parents spending more time with their children seem obvious. When spending more time with the child the parents will be able to inculcate healthy eating behaviors, and encourage the children to eat breakfast and to engage in physical activities.

Healthy habit formation in childhood is important for a child's later health (Livingstone et al. 2003; Malina 2001). While childhood obesity is in itself accompanied by serious health risks, overweight status is determined by the stock of net calories over the child's lifetime. The health consequences of an unhealthy lifestyle might therefore not show up in measurements of body weight until later in the child's life. Consequently, we focus on activities that are related to a healthy or an unhealthy lifestyle among children aged 7 to 17.

---

[1] Using a collective household production model with a two-stage Stackelberg game structure, in which the parents are the leaders and the child the follower, You and Davis (2010) show that childhood obesity is determined by several factors such as the amount and quality of food consumed at home and away from home, a child's time spent on exercise, and some biological, genetic and home environment factors.

The economic literature on childhood obesity hypothesizes that increased labor market participation among mothers leads to less time spent in the home (e.g. cooking, supervising and playing with the children) and more time during which children are unsupervised by their parents (Anderson et al. 2003a; Chia 2008; Ruhm 2008). Leaving children in the care of others or alone may have an impact on the children's eating habits and sedentary and physical activities if those who care for the children are less concerned about the children's health than are the parents, or if children tend to eat more calorie-dense food and engage more in sedentary activities when unsupervised.[2] Hence, studies from the US and Canada point toward a positive relationship between maternal employment and the time children spend watching television (Fertig et al. 2009; Chia 2008). Moreover, Chia (2008) shows a negative relationship between maternal employment and the time children spend on organized sport. Fertig et al. (2009) argue that the time children spend eating and the number of daily meals is related to overweight and obesity and find that maternal employment reduces occurrence of these activities.

This paper studies the relationship between parental working hours and parental child care time, as well as parental input into the production of children's health. In particular, we examine how the parent's own health behaviors are related to children's health behaviors, and we include not only the behavior of the mother but also that of the father, which is rarely done in the literature (Benson and Mokhtari, 2011).

Denmark makes an interesting context in which to study the relationship between children's lifestyles and both maternal and paternal employment. Given the high labor market participation among Danish mothers – one of the highest among the OECD countries – some of the decrease in mother-child time may be offset by an increase in Danish fathers' time with their children (OECD, 2001). In fact, Danish fathers spend more time on child care than fathers from, e.g. the US (24% more) and the UK (64% more) (Bonke, 2009).

The data used stem from the Danish time-use and Consumption Survey 2008/2009 (DTUC), which allows us to investigate the relationship between both maternal and paternal time use and children's everyday activities, i.e. whether breakfast is

---

[2] Several papers have examined the relationship between maternal employment and childhood obesity, where childhood obesity is measured by the body mass index, see Anderson et al. (2003b), Classen and Hokayem (2005), Fertig et al. (2009), Courtemanche (2009), Ruhm (2008) for U.S., Zhu (2007) for Australia, Phipps et al. (2006), Chia (2008) for Canada, Garcia et al. (2006) for Spain, Scholder (2008) for UK, and Greve (2011) for Denmark. Except for the Danish paper, all the other papers show that when mothers start working (more hours), their children are more likely to become overweight or obese.

eaten, the number of daily meals, and how much time children spend on exercise and TV/computer games referring to the numerous medical studies showing that children's lifestyles affect their current and future health outcomes.[3]

The main findings in the paper are that there is no relationship between maternal working hours and children's time allocations and lifestyles, and that paternal working hours are weakly associated with whether the child had breakfast. We find a significant relationship between parental working hours and child care, and find that parental child care matters for the children's everyday lives. Finally, estimations on the relationship between parental and children's time spent on exercise indicate that parental time use on healthy activities seems to be more relevant to children's lifestyle behavior than parental child care time.

2. Data

The Danish Time-Use and Consumption Survey (DTUC) was conducted over 12 months (March 2008-March 2009).[4] A sample of 6,000 people was drawn from administrative registers held by Statistics Denmark. The respondents first attended an interview which elicited basic information on, e.g. family relations and socioeconomic status. Respondents were then asked to complete two time-use diaries – one for a weekday and one for a weekend day – with 37 pre-coded activities (Table A1 provides a detailed description of the relevant activities). If respondents were between 18 and 74 years old and had a spouse or cohabiting partner and/or children aged 7-17, these other family members were also asked to complete two time-use diaries. If respondents had children aged 7-11, the parents were asked to assist them in completing the diary. The selected data set includes all families with children between 7 and 17 years of age.

Reporting of only the primary activity may have led to underreporting of certain other activities. For example, if some families ate meals while watching television, respondents had to decide which activity was the main activity. However, omitting television as a secondary activity is a minor problem, as this does not

---

[3] The dependent variables we examine are the number of meals eaten during the day, and if the child ate breakfast, both of which are inversely associated with childhood obesity up to a certain extent (Toscheke et al. 2009; Dubois et al. 2005). The other dependent variables are the children's time spent on television viewing, playing computer games and doing sport, which are considered good proxies for physical activities (Bittman et al. 2010), and related to both short- and long-term physical and mental health. (Penedo and Dahn 2005) and to obesity and lifestyle diseases (WHO 2004).

[4] A detailed description of DTUS is given in Bonke (2008), and an evaluation of the data quality is given in Bonke and Fallesen (2010).

necessarily displace time spent on other – non-sedentary – activities when it is the secondary activity.

With the help of a unique identifier, DTUC was merged with administrative register data enabling us to include register information on the interviewees in DTUC and to test for sample selection bias against the whole population, e.g. in the selected sample children with unemployed parents and children of immigrants are underrepresented. In this study, we used time-use information from 1,206 children living in 809 families. Because of the inclusion of siblings in the survey, we controlled for possible clustering effects.

Table 1 shows that the children (aged 7 to 17) had on average more than two meals per day, and that breakfast was eaten by 80% of the children (more often by the 7-11-year-olds than by the 12-17-year-olds) on a weekday. On average the children spent 32 minutes on exercise and 184 minutes on TV/computer games per day. Time spent on these activities differed significantly depending on the child's age, with the older children (12 to 17) spending more time on exercise and TV/computer games.

The figures for maternal and paternal working hours and child care are weighted averages of hours reported in the diaries for one weekday and one weekend day. As the diaries were collected on the same day for all family members, the actual time the parents spent away from or with the child refers to the same day the child carried out her/his activities. We found that mothers worked on average 3.6 hours and fathers on average 4.4 hours per day. The employment rates for the mothers and fathers participating in the survey were 93% and 96%, respectively.

The measure of parental time spent on child care is the number of minutes the parents spent on taking care of, helping, reading to and playing with their children. This means that time parents spent on activities in which the children were not directly involved – if the parents prepared meals while the child was playing in the kitchen – is not taken into account. The time parents spent on child care on a weighted day was on average 0.36 and 0.17 hours for mothers and fathers, respectively, with younger school children getting more care than older school children. Mothers spent on average 0.55 hours if the child was between 7 and 11 and 0.21 hours if the child was between 12 and 17, and fathers on average 0.26 versus 0.09 hours per day.

Table 1: Means and standard deviations in parentheses

	Full sample	7-11-yr-olds	12-17-yr-olds
Child activities			
– Number of meals	2.277	2.332	2.236
	(0.710)	(0.639)	(0.757)
– Breakfast (d)	0.808	0.866	0.763
	(0.394)	(0.341)	(0.426)
– Exercise	32.177	24.537	38.028
	(58.563)	(49.002)	(64.363)
– TV/computer games[a]	183.677	153.597	206.710
	(132.151)	(120.621)	(135.996)
Parental time use			
– Maternal working hours[a]	3.569	3.522	3.605
	(2.737)	(2.643)	(2.808)
– Maternal child care[a]	0.358	0.551	0.210
	(0.799)	(0.924)	(0.651)
– Paternal working hours[a]	4.390	4.402	4.380
	(3.194)	(3.185)	(3.203)
– Paternal child care[a]	0.166	0.261	0.093
	(0.378)	(0.462)	(0.277)
Maternal education			
– No post-secondary education	0.172	0.138	0.198
	(0.377)	(0.345)	(0.399)
– Vocational education	0.363	0.321	0.395
	(0.481)	(0.467)	(0.489)
– Short course tertiary education	0.046	0.052	0.041
	(0.209)	(0.221)	(0.198)
– Medium course tertiary education	0.315	0.371	0.272
	(0.465)	(0.484)	(0.445)
– Long course tertiary education	0.104	0.119	0.094
	(0.306)	(0.324)	(0.292)
Mother's age	42.086	39.579	44.006
	(5.103)	(4.462)	(4.719)
Age of child	12.111	9.096	14.420
	(3.080)	(1.407)	(1.713)

First-born child (d)	0.429	0.423	0.433
	(0.495)	(0.494)	(0.496)
Child below 7 in HH (d)	0.217	0.371	0.100
	(0.503)	(0.610)	(0.362)
Boy (d)	0.533	0.545	0.524
	(0.499)	(0.498)	(0.500)
Non-normal school day (d)	0.284	0.254	0.307
	(0.451)	(0.436)	(0.462)
N	1206	523	683

Note: The sample is restricted to families with at least one child between 7 and 17 years of age in the household. a: time-use variables are weighted averages for one weekday and one weekend day. (d) dummy variable.

Parental education refers to the longest completed course of education: no post-secondary education, vocational training, short-course tertiary education (less than 3 years), medium-course tertiary education (3 to 4 years), and long-course tertiary education (more than 4 years). To avoid multicollinearity we left out measures of paternal education in the estimations, as the lengths of paternal and maternal education are correlated. Net annual household income (in quantiles) is included in the analyses to correct for variation in consumption possibilities.

Additional control variables are child's age and gender, whether the child was the first-born, whether there was a child below 6 in the family, mother's age, whether the child's weekday was a non-normal school day, and area of residence (metropolis, urban or rural).

3. The empirical strategy

To estimate the relationship between parents' time with their children and their children's time use and other health-related variables, we estimated a single model for each outcome. The time-use outcomes and number of meals are weighted averages of a weekday and a weekend day. Due to the distribution of the different outcomes, we present OLS results when estimating number of daily meals, time spent on exercise and time spent on TV/computer games.[5] We present probit models for the outcome whether or not the child ate breakfast.

---

[5] We have also estimated ordered probit models for the number of meals. However, the results from the ordered probit models were virtually the same as for the OLS models. For simplicity we present the OLS results; the ordered probit results are available upon request.

Although variables measuring time spent on exercise and TV/computer games have a significant number of zero minutes, zero minutes spent on these activities do not necessarily imply that the child never engages in these activities. OLS regressions were therefore chosen because they estimate time-use data better than Tobit and two-part models (Stewart 2009).

Identifying the causal relationship between parental time use and that of their children is difficult, because parents' decisions to spend time with their children may also be determined by the children's lifestyles: children with preferences for sport may spend a significant amount of their time in a sports club, for which reason the parents may spend less time with their children, and perhaps decide to work more hours. Parental time use on children may also be determined by unobserved factors, such as time preferences that directly affect the outcome. To take this into account, we used instrumental variables to test for exogeneity in the variables measuring maternal and paternal working hours.

The instruments we used to test for exogeneity in parental working hours were: the grandmothers' employment status when the mother and father were 16 years old, and information on local taxes in 271 municipalities in Denmark, controlling for education and income effects.[6] While the grandmothers' employment status influences parental, especially maternal, working hours, it does not exert direct influence on the children's activities. The municipal tax rate is set annually by the local authorities on the basis of estimated municipal expenses within government-set limits for tax differences between municipalities. Consequently, the tax rate is expected to have an impact on the supply of parental labor but to be unrelated to how each child spends his or her time. However, in the first stage regression, the F-statistic of the instruments, we found that the best sets of instruments were grandmothers' employment for maternal working hours and grandmothers' employment and municipal tax rates for paternal working hours. The F-statistic was right above 2 in both regressions, indicating that the selected instruments are relatively weak.[7] As the models could not converge with two endogenous variables, the IV regressions we estimated included only either maternal or paternal working hours as endogenous. We tested the results from the IV models with a Davidson and MacKinnon (1993) test in the linear models and a Wald test in the non-linear models, and we found that we cannot reject maternal and paternal working hours as being exogenous. These results are available on request.

---

[6] The tax rates varied between 22.1 and 27.5 with a mean of 24.9 and standard deviation of 0.79.

[7] Different sets of instruments have been tested. For example, the F-statistic is above 2 when only the grandmother's employment is used on maternal working hours and the local tax rate is used on paternal working hours.

4. Results

4.1 Parental working time and child care time

Table 2 presents correlation coefficients between parental working hours and child care.[8] The correlation coefficients show the expected negative relationship between maternal employment and child care. However, this relationship is only significant among mothers with children aged 7 to 11 and is relatively small and far from being a one-to-one relationship. For fathers with children aged 12 to 17 the correlation between employment and child care is positive and significant, but again relatively small. We also find a positive, but small and insignificant, relationship between maternal employment and paternal child care and between paternal employment and maternal child care (the latter being significant for the 12-17-years-olds).

Table 2: Descriptive statistics, correlation coefficients between parental time spent on paid work and child care.

	Mother's working hours	Father's working hours
Full sample, N=1206		
– Mother's working hours	-	0.26*
– Father's working hours	0.26*	-
– Mother's child care	-0.09*	0.037
– Father's child care	0.001	0.057*
7-11-year-olds, N=523		
– Mother's working hours	-	0.27*
– Father's working hours	0.27*	-
– Mother's child care	-0.12*	0.002
– Father's child care	-0.006	0.03
12-17-year-olds, N=683		
– Mother's working hours	-	0.25
– Father's working hours	0.25	-
– Mother's child care	-0.07	0.08*
– Father's child care	0.02	0.09*

All variables are weighted average for a weekday and a weekend day.
  Notes: *: Significant at 5%. The sample is restricted to families with at least one child in the household between 7 and 17 years of age.

---

[8] Note that among mothers and fathers respectively 30% and 26% report no working hours and 56% and 70% report no child care time.

4.2 Parental working time and children's activities

In previous literature parental working time has been used as a measure of time input into the child health production function. Table 3 presents the results on the relationship between parental working hours (on a weighted day) and children's activities for the full sample. We find that maternal working hours are not significantly related to any of the children's activities, while the father's work is negatively correlated (10% level) with his child's breakfast behavior: if the father is working one more hour a day the child is 1% less likely to eat breakfast on a weekday.

Children's activities are strongly related to their age, as older children have fewer meals, eat breakfast less often, watch more television and participate more in sports than do younger children. Estimating the same models for a sample of 7-11- and 12--17-year-olds, respectively, we came up with virtually identical results (not shown).

If one of the reported days is a non-normal school day (the child is not at school) it is less likely that s/he eats breakfast, and the number of meals in general goes down while time spent on TV/computer games goes up. If the mother has a long-course higher education compared to no post-secondary education, the child spends more time on exercise and less time on TV/computer games. The child is also more likely to eat breakfast on a weekday when the mother has a long-course higher education than when she has no post-secondary education. The relationship between higher household income and the time the child spends on TV/computer games is negative, while boys are more likely than girls to spend time on exercise and on TV/computer games.

Table 3: Parental working hours and child activities.

	#Meals	Breakfast	Exercise	TV/computer
Maternal working hours	-0.00485	0.000896	0.781	0.451
	(-0.55)	(0.21)	(1.02)	(0.28)
Paternal working hours	0.00125	-0.00633+	-0.260	2.106
	(0.16)	(-1.70)	(-0.43)	(1.56)
Non-normal school day	-0.151**	-0.437***	2.175	42.20***
	(-2.86)	(-13.11)	(0.48)	(4.07)
Vocational education	0.0641	0.0386	4.986	-5.526
	(0.94)	(1.28)	(0.89)	(-0.48)

Short course tertiary education	0.0776	0.0538	-1.632	11.29
	(0.73)	(1.22)	(-0.20)	(0.55)
Medium course tertiary education	-0.00592	0.0453	1.342	-20.12+
	(-0.08)	(1.46)	(0.23)	(-1.67)
Long course tertiary education	0.115	0.0608+	15.70*	-26.55+
	(1.16)	(1.89)	(1.98)	(-1.69)
Mother's age	0.00769	0.000193	0.246	1.509
	(1.26)	(0.07)	(0.58)	(1.62)
Boy	-0.0519	0.0135	5.747+	40.01***
	(-1.25)	(0.64)	(1.66)	(5.20)
Child below 7 in HH	-0.00616	-0.0165	-4.857	-9.564
	(-0.14)	(-0.57)	(-1.59)	(-0.98)
Age of child (12-17/7-11)	-0.0216**	-0.0147***	1.258*	5.943***
	(-2.60)	(-3.42)	(2.11)	(4.05)
HH income, 2nd quantile	-0.00355	0.0208	4.981	-15.26
	(-0.05)	(0.64)	(0.91)	(-1.22)
HH income, 3rd quantile	0.0217	0.000156	1.043	-16.69
	(0.31)	(0.00)	(0.19)	(-1.30)
HH income, 4th quantile	-0.0823	0.00422	0.568	-22.22+
	(1.11)	(0.12)	(0.10)	(-1.68)
Adj./Pseudo R^2	0.010	0.25	0.008	0.086

OLS estimate for number of meals, time spent on exercise and on TV/computer games. Probit estimation (marginal effects) for breakfast at weekdays. Number of observations = 1206.

Notes: t statistics in parentheses. + p<0.10, * p<0.05, ** p<0.01, *** p<0.001. The sample is restricted to families with at least one child in the household between 7 and 17 years of age.

Whether the child was the first-born in family and dummy variables for area of residence are included but not shown.

Models, corresponding to the results in Table 3, were estimated using the parents' aggregate working hours and the paternal share of total parental working hours. Furthermore, the models were estimated omitting paternal and maternal working hours separately. These results did not, however, add more information to the results shown in Table 3. The results are available on request.

4.3 Parental child care time and children's activities

Table 4 presents results from the estimated relationship between parental child care time and children's activities. Additional control variables have been left out of the table, because the parameter estimates are nearly the same as the parameter estimates shown in Table 3. The estimation on the full sample shows a negative relationship between parental child care and the child's time spent on TV/computer games: a 1-hour increase in maternal and paternal child care time decreases the child's time spent on TV/computer games by 12 and 19 minutes, respectively. Among 7-11-year-olds maternal child care is associated with more children having breakfast and more time spent on exercise. Paternal child care is associated with less time spent on exercise and less time spent on TV/computer games. While paternal child care does not seem to be significantly related with children's activities among 12-17-year-olds, maternal child care is associated with less time spent on exercise and on TV/computer games.

While parental child care time seems to be a contributing factor to children's health behavior activities, the explained variance only changed slightly when including parental child care time in the models explaining number of meals, breakfast and time spent on exercise. The R^2 in the models estimating the number of meals was 0.012 without parental child care time included and 0.011 when parental child care time was included. For the models estimating time spent on exercise the R^2's were 0.009 and 0.008, and in the models estimating time spent on TV/computer games the R^2 were 0.085 and 0.091 without and with parental child care, respectively.

Table 4: Parental child care and child activities.

	#Meals	Breakfast	Exercise	TV/computer
Full sample				
Maternal child care	0.0141	0.0170	1.692	-11.85**
	(0.41)	(0.99)	(0.82)	(-2.60)
Paternal child care	0.0689	0.0593	-5.808	-18.86*
	(1.21)	(1.33)	(-1.57)	(-2.07)
N	1206	1206	1206	1206
Adj./Pseudo R^2	0.011	0.25	0.008	0.091
7 to 11 years of age				
Maternal child care	-0.00821	0.0373*	7.330**	-6.062
	(-0.20)	(2.04)	(2.83)	(-1.24)
Paternal child care	0.0864	0.0335	-10.11**	-20.49*
	(1.36)	(0.95)	(-2.98)	(-2.14)

N	523	523	523	523
Adj./Pseudo R²	-0.001	0.23	0.038	0.131
12 to 17 years of age				
Maternal child care	0.0633	-0.00178	-4.755*	-14.20**
	(1.48)	(-0.07)	(-2.06)	(-2.66)
Paternal child care	0.0276	0.0940	1.845	-17.79
	(0.26)	(1.06)	(0.21)	(-1.12)
N	683	683	683	683
Adj./Pseudo R²	0.014	0.27	0.004	0.067

OLS estimation for number of meals, time spent on exercise and on TV/computer games. Probit estimation (marginal effects) for breakfast at weekdays.

Notes: Marginal effects; t statistics in parentheses. + p<0.10, * p<0.05, ** p<0.01, *** p<0.001. The sample is restricted to families with at least one child in the household between 7 and 17 years of age. All estimations include the following control variables: age of mother, child's gender, child's age, whether the child is the eldest child in the family, whether there is a child below 6 years of age in the household, maternal education, household income, whether it was a non-normal school day and dummy variables for area of residence.

4.4 Parental activities and child activities

In Table 5 we included measures of parental behavior instead of parental time use while including the same control variables as in the previous estimations. This means that when we estimated the model on the time a child spent on exercise, we included parental time spent on exercise.

We find that for the full sample parental activities became significant in nearly all the models, the exception being the coefficient for the relationship between mother and child breakfast, which was not significant. The results differ when we estimate the models separately for children aged 7-11 and 12-17. Among younger children the results show a positive relationship between parental and children's behavior. However, the results for paternal number of meals, doing exercise and time spent on TV/computer games were only significant at 10%, and for maternal time spent on exercise we found no significant correlation with the child's time spent on exercise.

For children aged 12-17 the relationships between paternal and maternal, and child time spent on TV/computer games were not significant. Furthermore, paternal behaviors: whether the father ate breakfast, the number of meals he had, and the time he spent on exercise were positive and significantly related to the same child activities. When the father spends one hour more on exercise, the child spends 11.4 more minutes on exercise. For mothers of older children, the size of the parameter estimate for maternal time spent on exercise is 12.4, but the result is only significant at 10%. For number of meals, eating breakfast, and looking at TV/computer games there were no significant relationship between maternal and child behavior.

Table 5: Parental activities and child activities, and different control variablses.[1]

	#Meals	Breakfast	Exercise	TV/computer
Full sample				
Mother, meals	0.0877**			
	(3.19)			
Father, meals	0.0981***			
	(3.89)			
Mother, breakfast		0.0390		
		(1.46)		
Father, breakfast		0.0857**		
		(3.17)		
Mother, exercise			9.248**	
			(2.63)	
Father, exercise			9.814**	
			(2.88)	
Mother, TV/ computer				9.702**
				(2.93)
Father, TV/computer				5.724*
				(2.37)
N	1206	1206	1206	1206
Adj./Pseudo R^2	0.041		0.040	0.101
7 to 11 years of age				
Mother, meals	0.120**			
	(2.94)			
Father, meals	0.0628+			
	(1.77)			
Mother, breakfast		0.0483+		
		(1.71)		
Father, breakfast		0.0701*		
		(2.49)		
Mother, exercise			4.288	
			(1.14)	

Father, exercise			9.166+	
			(1.67)	
Mother, TV/ computer				15.19***
				(3.33)
Father, TV/computer				5.216+
				(1.76)
N	523	523	523	523
Adj./Pseudo R^2	0.028		0.044	0.157
12 to 17 years of age				
Mother, meals	0.0534			
	(1.48)			
Father, meals	0.127***			
	(3.82)			
Mother, breakfast		0.00989		
		(0.25)		
Father, breakfast		0.0818*		
		(2.03)		
Mother, exercise			12.40+	
			(1.76)	
Father, exercise			11.40**	
			(2.66)	
Mother, TV/ computer				7.079
				(1.64)
Father, TV/computer				5.005
				(1.57)
N	683	683	683	683
Adj./Pseudo R^2	0.045		0.041	0.071

OLS estimation for number of meals, time spent on exercise and on TV/computer games. Probit estimation (marginal effects) for breakfast at weekdays.

Notes: Marginal effects; t statistics in parentheses. + $p<0.10$, * $p<0.05$, ** $p<0.01$, *** $p<0.001$. The sample is restricted to families with at least one child in the household between 7 and 17 years of age.

[1] Age of mother, child's gender, child's age, whether the child is the eldest child in the family, whether there is a child below 6 years of age in the household, maternal education, household income, whether it was a non-normal school day and dummy variables for area of residence.

Compared to basis models without parental time or behavioral characteristics the models in which parental behavior was included increased the explained variance significantly. For example, the R^2 increased from 0.012 to 0.041 in the model estimating number of meals, from 0.009 to 0.040 in the model estimating time spent on exercise and from 0.085 to 0.101 in the model estimating time spent on TV/computer games.

5. Conclusions

According to medical literature later consequences of unhealthy lifestyle behaviors can be traced back to the lifestyle behaviors the individual had at school age (Livingstone et al. 2003; Malina 2001). Consequently, this paper focuses on how parents can influence their children's health and lifestyle behavior when they are aged 7 to 17.

We use a Danish time use and consumption survey from 2008/2009, which includes time use information from all family members above 7 years of age, merged with Danish register data, to study the relationship between parental time and behavior and their children's everyday activities, i.e. whether breakfast is eaten, the number of daily meals, and how much time children spend on exercise, TV/computer games.

Applying different statistical estimations the present study examined the relationship between both maternal and paternal working time on their children's lifestyle behavior. As opposed to investigations for other countries, we found no significant relationship between maternal working hours and children's unhealthy activities and only a weak negative relationship between paternal working hours and whether the child ate breakfast.

Although there have been changing time-use patterns in Danish families due to an increase in women's labor market participation, this does not mean that parents spend less time with their children. Thus, Bonke (2009) finds that the time Danish parents spent with their children on weekdays increased from 1 hour 18 minutes in 1987 to 1 hour 49 minutes in 2008. Simple correlations between parental time spent on working and parental time spent on child care showed that maternal working hours were negatively correlated with maternal child care (among children aged 7-11), while paternal working hours were positively correlated with paternal child care (among children aged 12-17). However, the correlation coefficients are relatively small, suggesting that parental employment is not a good proxy of parental child care time.

The associations between parental child care and children's activities exhibited a significant relationship. We found that maternal child care was associated with a higher probability of the child having breakfast and more time spent on exercise for children aged 7 to 11. For children aged 12 to 17, maternal child care was associated with less time spent on exercise and on TV/computer games. The negative relationship between maternal child care and exercise for this group seems to indicate that children of this age are more likely to spend time away from home and less likely to spend time with their mother when they join sports clubs, etc.

Paternal child care seems to be associated with less time spent on exercise and TV/computer games for children aged 7 to 11. These results indicate that it is mainly the mother, not the father, who takes the children (aged 7 to 11) to sports activities while an increase in both maternal and paternal child care reduces the child's time spent on TV/computer games.

While parental child care is associated with children's lifestyle behavior, the explained variance from including the parental child care time in the models only slightly changed the explained variance, suggesting that parental child care time might not be the most important way in which parents can influence their children's lifestyle. Instead, when we included the parents' time use on the relevant child lifestyle behavior, these variables were in most cases significantly associated with the children's behavior and the explained variance increased significantly in all models.

These results suggest that parental behavior is important for the child to develop a healthy lifestyle. Future research to obtain a detailed understanding of how parents can influence their children's lifestyles and health needs to leave the focus only on maternal working time. Instead this study has shown the relevance of not only including maternal but also paternal characteristics, and stressed that parental inputs into the child health production function, such as the parents own health behavior, might be important for the children to develop a healthy lifestyle that will form the basis of their future health.

References

Anderson, P., Butcher, K.F. & Levine, P.B. (2003a). Maternal employment and overweight children. *Journal of Health Economics*, 22, 477-504.

Anderson, P., Butcher, K.F. & Levine, P.B. (2003b). Economic perspectives on childhood obesity. *Economic Perspectives*. 3Q, 30-48.

Benson, L & M. Mokhtari (2011). Parental Employment, Shared Parent-Child Activities and Childhood Obesity. *Journal of Family Economic issues* 32, 233-244.

Bonke, J. (2008). *Project proposal. An investigation of time-use and consumption within Danish families, with special emphasis on children*. Rockwool Foundation Research Unit.

Bonke, J. & P. Fallesen (2010).The impact of incentives and interview methods on response quantity and quality in diary and booklet based surveys. *Survey Research Methods*. 4(2), 91-101.

Bonke, J. & Greve, J (2010). *Health, Well-being and overweight in Denmark* (Danish title: Helbred, trivsel og overvægt blandt danskere). Gyldendal, Copenhagen, Denmark.

Bonke, J. (2009). *Parental child care and money spent on their children (In Danish)*. Rockwool Foundation Research Unit and University Press of Southern Denmark.

Chia, Y. F. 2008. Maternal Labour Supply and Childhood Obesity in Canada: Evidence from the NLSCY. *Canadian Journal of Economics* 41(1), 217-242.

Chou S. Y., Grossman, M. & Saffer, H. (2002). An economic analysis of adult obesity: results from the Behavioral Risk Factor Surveillance System. NBER working paper 9247.

Classen, T., C. Hokayem. 2005. Childhood influences on youth obesity. Economics and Human Biology, 3:165-87.

Courtemanche, C. 2009. Longer Hours and Larger Waistlines? The Relationship between Work Hours and Obesity. Forum for Health Economics & Policy, 12, 2.

Cutler, D, Glaeser, E.L. & Shapiro, J. M. (2003). Why Have Americans Become More Obese? *Journal of Economic Perspectives.* 17(3), 93-118.

Davidson R. & MacKinnon, J. G. (1993) *Estimation and Inference in Econometrics.* Oxford University Press, New York.

Dubois, L., Girad, M. & Kent, M.P. (2005). Eating breakfast and overweight in pre-school population: Is there a link? *Public Health Nutrition*, 9(4), 436-442.

Ebbelin, C.B., Rawlak, D.B.& Ludwig, D.S. (2002). Childhood obesity: public-health crisis, common sense cure. *The Lancet*, 360, 473-482.

Fertig, A., G. Glomm & R. Tchernis. (2009). The connection between maternal employment and childhood obesity: inspecting the mechanism. *Review of Economics of the Household*, 7, 227-255.

Garcia, E., J. Labeaga, and C. Ortega. 2006. Maternal employment and childhood obesity in Spain. Working Paper FEDEA, Madrid.

Greve, Jane (2011); "New Results on the Effect of Maternal Work Hours on Children's Overweight Status: Does the Quality of Child Care Matter?". Labour Economics.

Kiens, B, Beyer, N., Brage, S., Hyldstrup, L., Ottesen, L. S., Overgaards, K., Pedersen, B. K., Puggaard, L. (2007) Consequences of a physically inactive lifestyle (Fysisk inaktivitet – konsekvenser og sammenhænge) Motions- og ernæringsrådet nr 3. Retrieved from: http://www.meraadet.dk/gfx/uploads/rapporter_pdf/13.06.07%207767_fysisk_inaktivitet_webny2.pdf

Lean, M, Lara, J., Hill, J. O. (2006). ABC of obesity. Strategies for preventing obesity. *BMJ*, 333, 959-962.

Livinstone, M. B., Robson, P.J., Wallance, J.M.,& McKinley, M.C. (2003) Proc. Nutr. Soc. 62 (3), 681-701.

Malina, R. M. (2001). Physical activity and fitness: pathways from childhood to adulthood. *Am. J. Hum. Biol.* 13(2), 162-172.

OECD (2001). Early Childhood Education and Care Policies in Denmark. OECD country note.

Phipps, Shelly A., Lynn Lethbridge, and Peter Burton. 2006. Long-run consequences of parental paid work hours for child overweight status in Canada. Social Science & Medicine, 62: 977-986.

Ruhm, C. J. (2008). Maternal employment and adolescent development. *Labour Economics,* 15(5), 958-983.

Scholder, Stephanie von Hinke Kessler. 2008. Maternal Employment and Overweight Children: Does Timing Matter? Health Economics 17: 889-906.

Stewart, J. (2009). Tobit or Not Tobit?, Bureau of Labor Statistics. Working Paper No. 432, November 2009.

World Health Organization. WHO (2004). Global Strategy on Diet, Physical Activity, and Health. Retrieved from: http://www.who.int/dietphysicalactivity/strategy/eb11344/strategy_english_web.pdf

You, W. & Davis, G. C. (2010). Household Food Expenditures, Parental Time Allocation, and Childhood Overweight: An Integrated Two-Stage Collective Model with an Empirical Application and Test. *American Journal of Agricultural Economics* 92(3), 849-858.

Zhu, A. 2007. The Effect of Maternal Employment on the Likelihood of a Child Being Overweight. Discussion Paper 2007/17, School of Economics, University of New South Wales.

Appendix

Table A1: Definition of children's activities

Activities	HETUS-2000 codes	Description
Paid work	111, 121	Working time in main job, working time in second job
Child care	38, 938	Child care, transporting a child
Exercise/sport	610, 611-617, 619	Physical activity, playing ball games, roller-skating, etc.
TV7computer games	821-822, 722-725	TV and video/DVD, PlayStation/computer games/Internet
Meals	010-011, 012, 531	Eating sessions
Eating breakfast	010-011, 012, 531	Eating session within 90 min. after a night's sleep between 05:30 and 11:00

Acknowledgements

The paper was presented at SFI – The National Centre for Social Research, at IATUR 2009 in Lunenburg, and at ESPE 2010 in Essen. We thank the participants at these presentations for their comments; we also thank Nabanita Datta Gupta, John Cawley, and Jay Stewart and the referees for valuable comments on previous drafts of the paper.